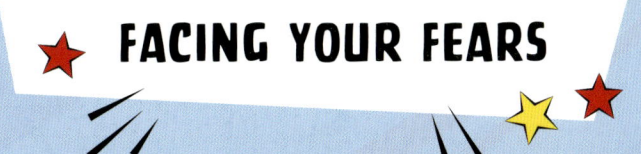

FACING YOUR FEAR OF VACCINATIONS

BY HEATHER E. SCHWARTZ

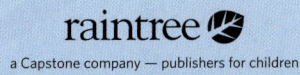

a Capstone company — publishers for children

Raintree is an imprint of Capstone Global Library Limited, a company incorporated in England and Wales having its registered office at 264 Banbury Road, Oxford, OX2 7DY – Registered company number: 6695582

www.raintree.co.uk
myorders@raintree.co.uk

Hardback edition © Capstone Global Library Limited 2023
Paperback edition © Capstone Global Library Limited 2024
The moral rights of the proprietor have been asserted.

All rights reserved. No part of this publication may be reproduced in any form or by any means (including photocopying or storing it in any medium by electronic means and whether or not transiently or incidentally to some other use of this publication) without the written permission of the copyright owner, except in accordance with the provisions of the Copyright, Designs and Patents Act 1988 or under the terms of a licence issued by the Copyright Licensing Agency, 5th Floor, Shackleton House, 4 Battle Bridge Lane, London SE1 2HX (www.cla.co.uk). Applications for the copyright owner's written permission should be addressed to the publisher.

Edited by Donald Lemke
Designed by Sarah Bennett
Original illustrations © Capstone Global Library Limited 2023
Picture research by Julie DeAdder
Production by Katy LaVigne
Originated by Capstone Global Library Ltd

978 1 3982 4883 0 (hardback)
978 1 3982 4882 3 (paperback)

British Library Cataloguing in Publication Data
A full catalogue record for this book is available from the British Library.

Acknowledgements
We would like to thank the following for permission to reproduce photographs: Getty Images: Dejan Dundjerski, 5, FatCamera, 15, JGI/Tom Grill, 18, omgimages, 19, SDI Productions, cover, 9, 13, Sean Justice, 12, ViewStock, 14; Shutterstock: Davizro Photography, 10, Domira (background), cover and throughout, Kapitosh (cloud), cover and throughout, Marish (brave girl), cover and throughout, Monkey Business Images, 4, New Africa, 8, Olena Yakobchuk, 17, paulaphoto, 11, Peakstock, 21, photastic, 20, Prostock-studio, 16, TinnaPong, 7

Every effort has been made to contact copyright holders of material reproduced in this book. Any omissions will be rectified in subsequent printings if notice is given to the publisher.

All the internet addresses (URLs) given in this book were valid at the time of going to press. However, due to the dynamic nature of the internet, some addresses may have changed, or sites may have changed or ceased to exist since publication. While the author and publisher regret any inconvenience this may cause readers, no responsibility for any such changes can be accepted by either the author or the publisher.

Printed and bound in India

CONTENTS

Scared of vaccinations.............................. 4

All about vaccinations 6

Needles are needed 10

After a vaccination 16

    Help a fuzzy friend 20

    Glossary 22

    Find out more 23

    Index 24

    About the author 24

Words in **bold** are in the glossary.

SCARED OF VACCINATIONS

Lots of children fear going to the doctor for one reason. They don't like vaccinations. Just the idea of getting one may make you worry.

But vaccinations are important. Learning more about them can help you feel calmer at the doctor's surgery.

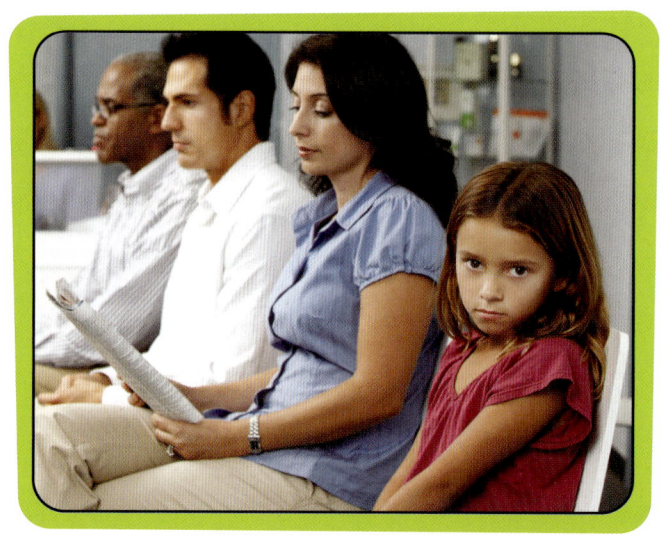

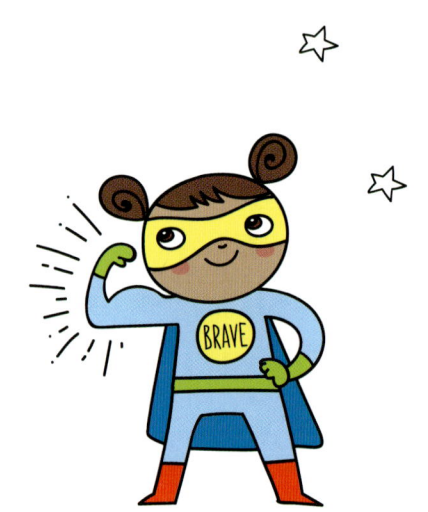

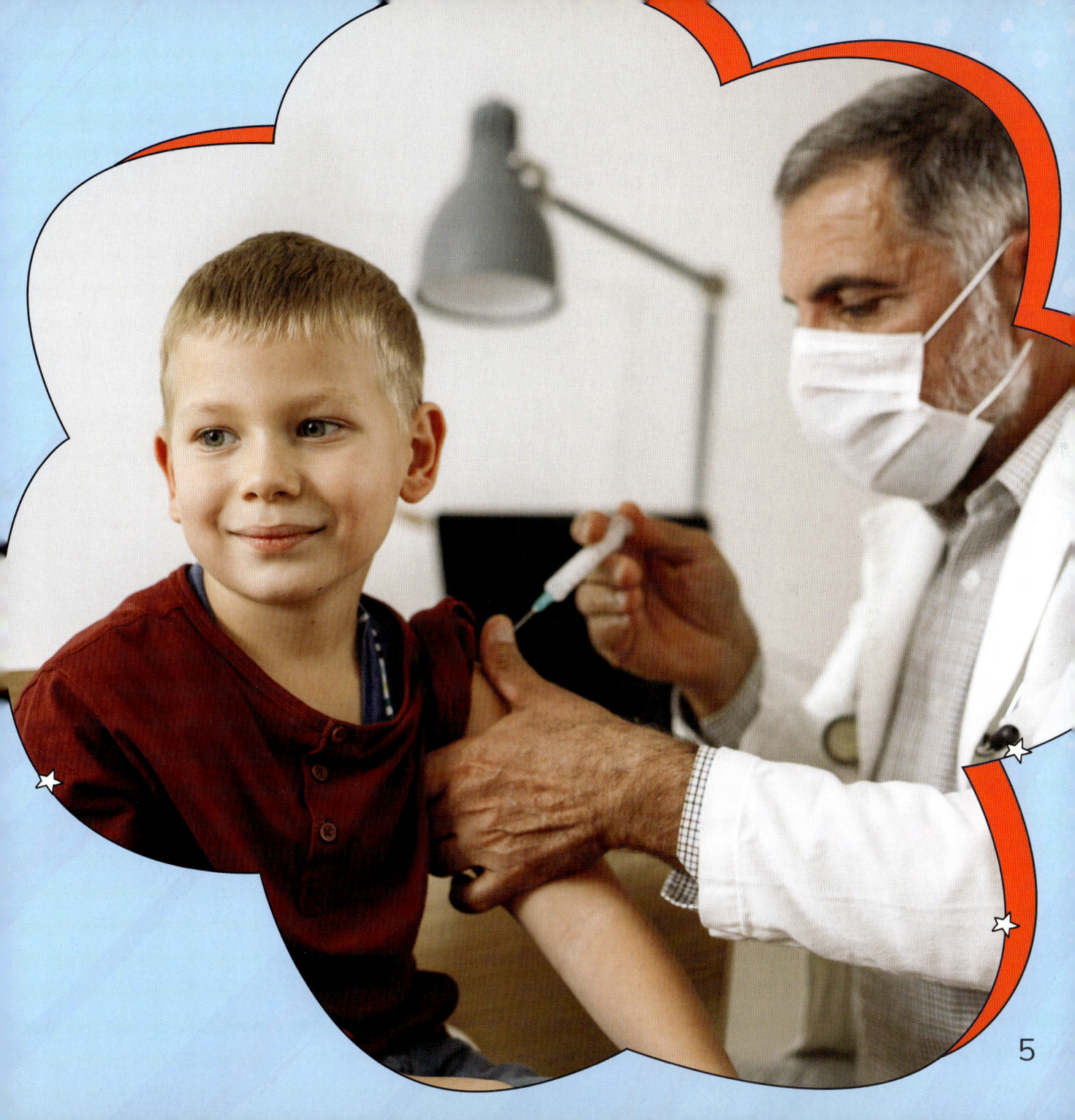

ALL ABOUT VACCINATIONS

Do you ever wish that vaccinations didn't exist? Then you wouldn't have to think about them. You would never have to get them.

But vaccinations are good for you. They help to keep you healthy. They teach your body how to fight **illnesses**.

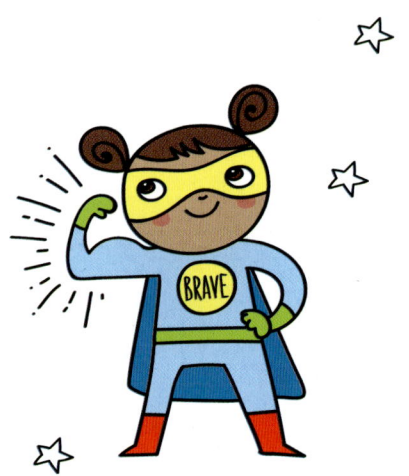

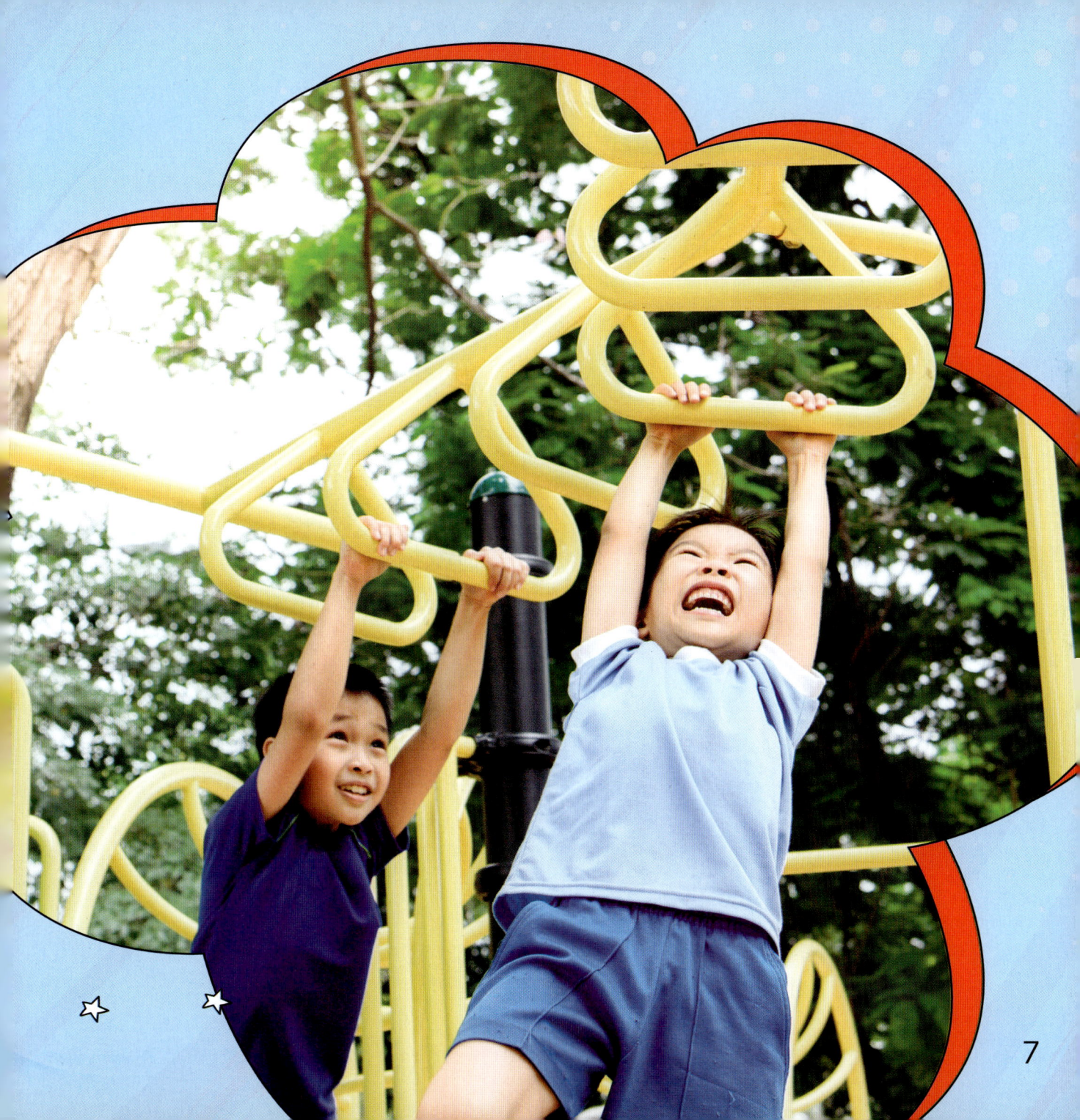

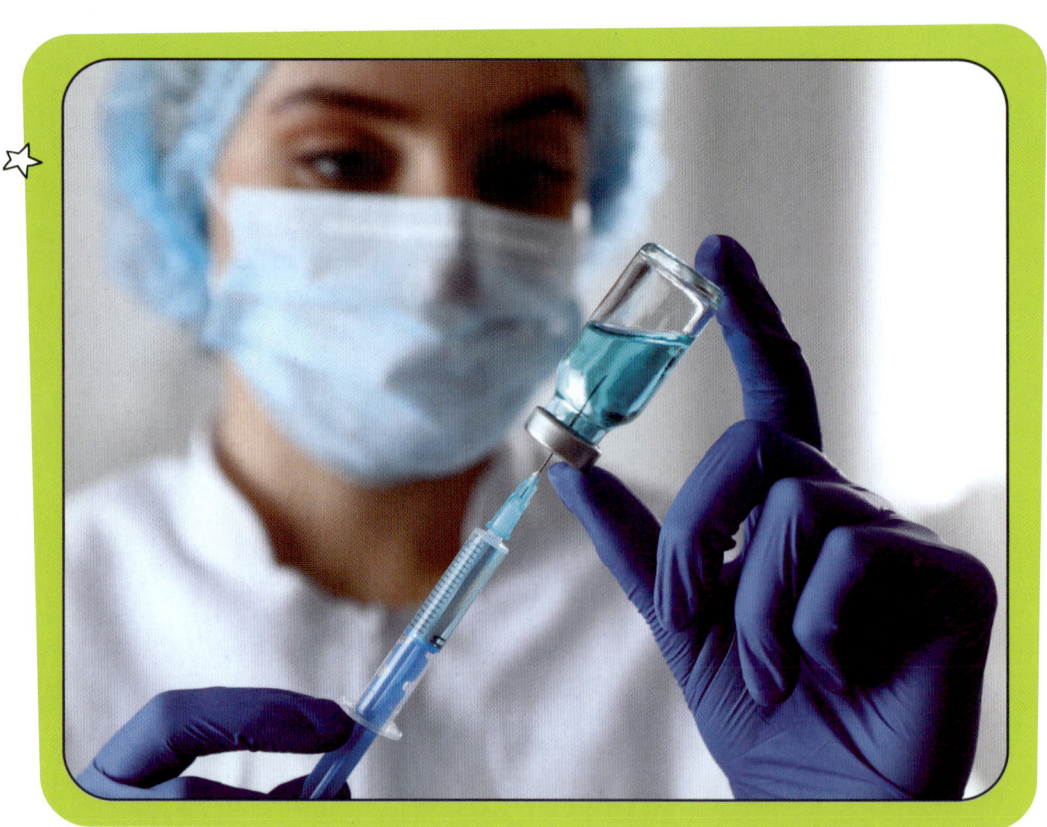

Injections deliver **vaccines**. Vaccines teach your body how to fight diseases. Some vaccines do this by using a weak or dead **virus** that won't make you ill.

After a vaccine, your body knows how to fight the virus. Your **immune system** can beat the disease and keep you well.

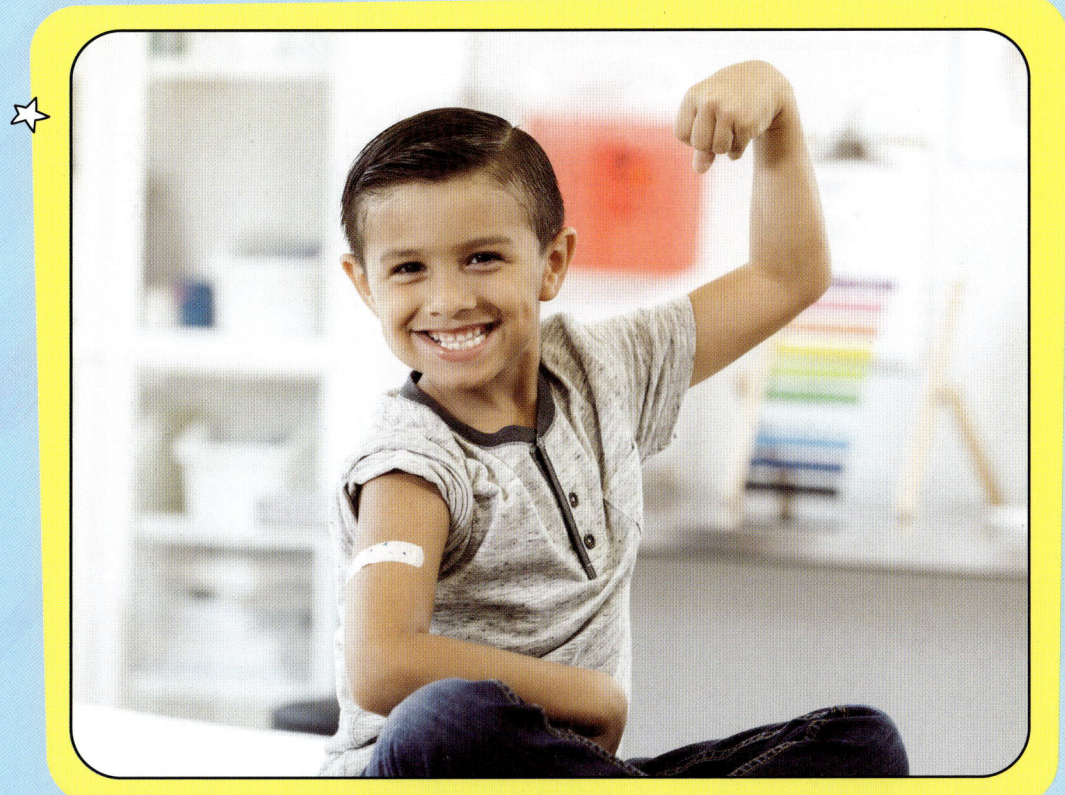

NEEDLES ARE NEEDED

Vaccines get into your body through a needle. Some people dislike needles. But not everyone does. You don't have to be afraid just because other people feel fearful.

Try this trick to calm down. Ask yourself: "Am I scared of needles?" Maybe the answer will surprise you. Maybe you are not afraid of them.

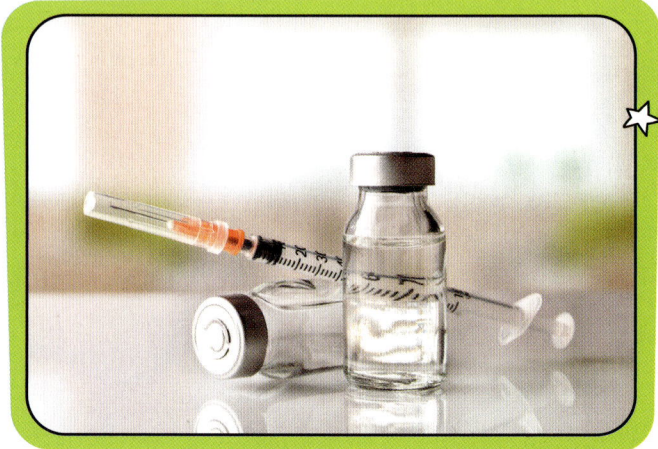

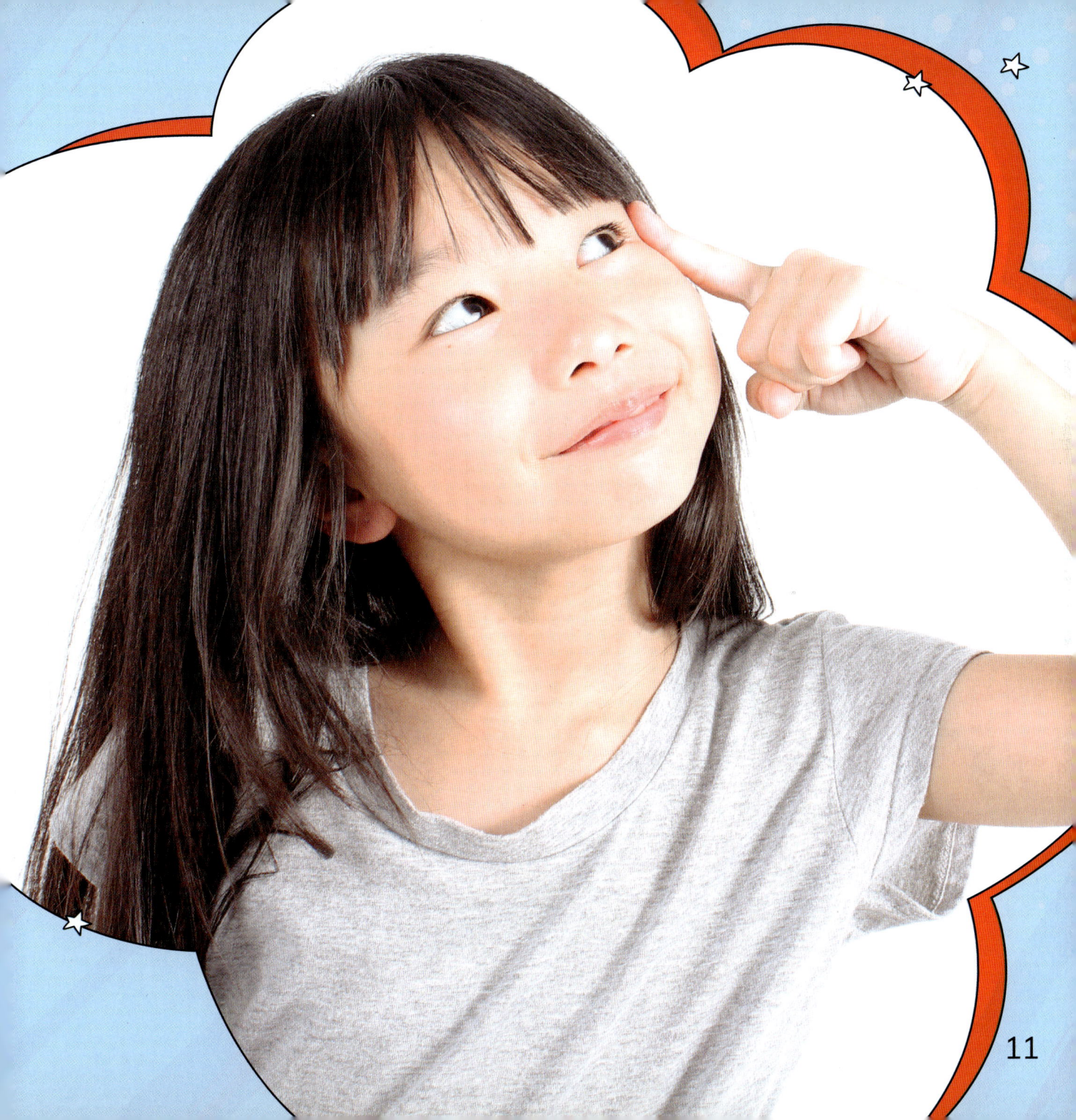

Vaccinations are easier to deal with if you can relax. One way to do that is by not thinking about them.

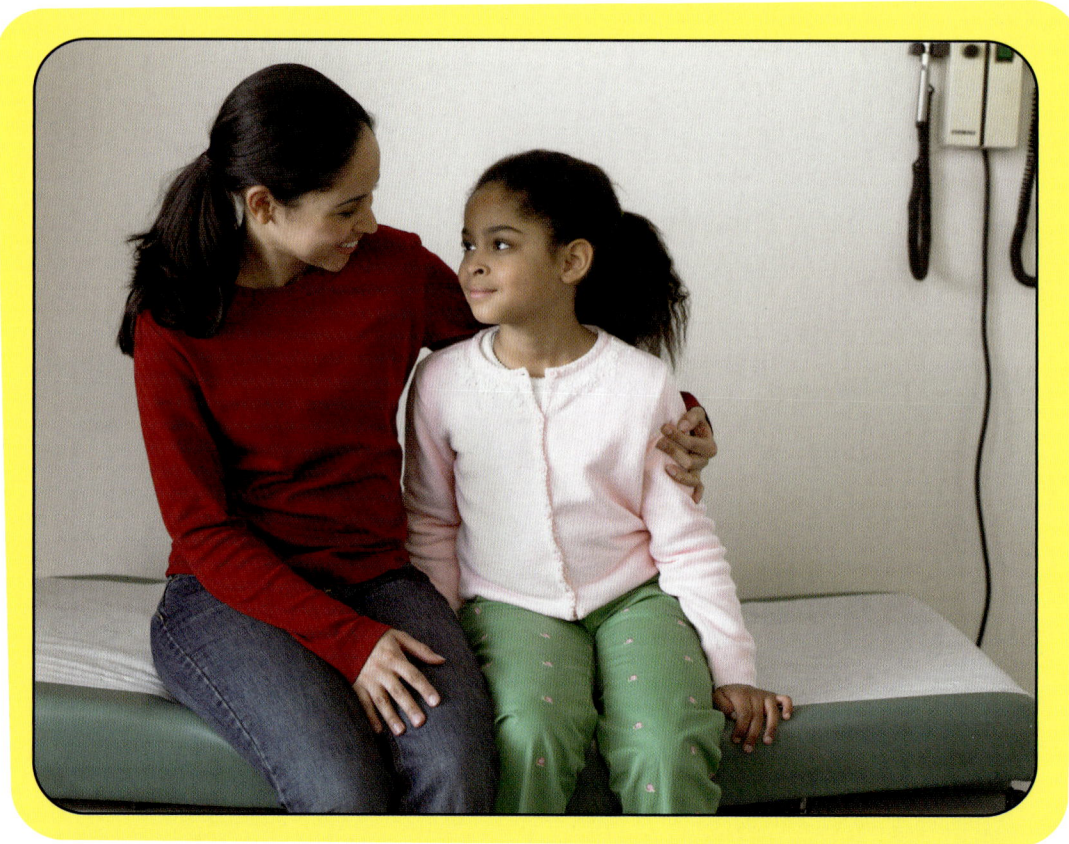

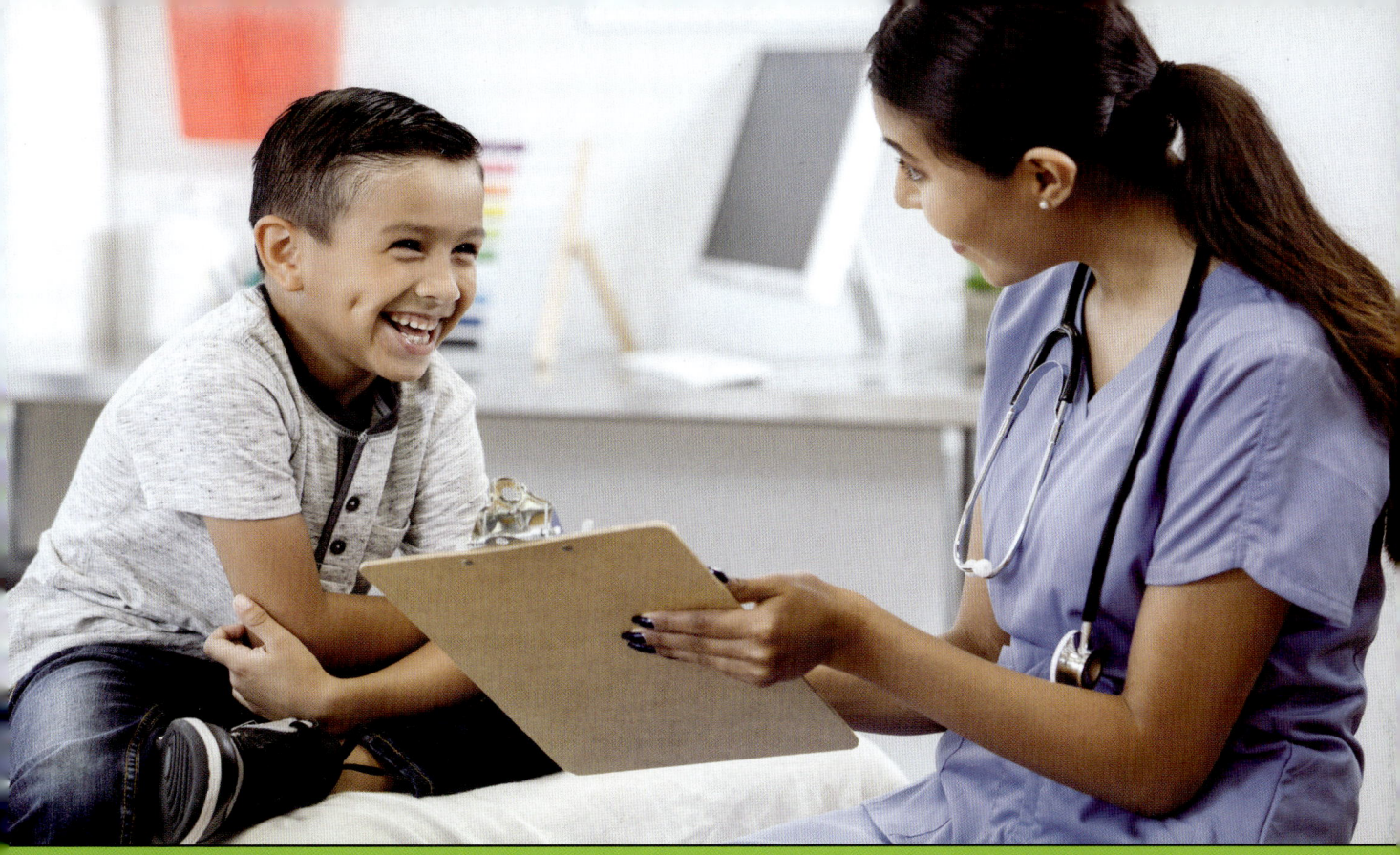

When it's time for a vaccination, focus your mind on a happy memory. **Distract** yourself by singing a song. Try telling a joke to the nurse.

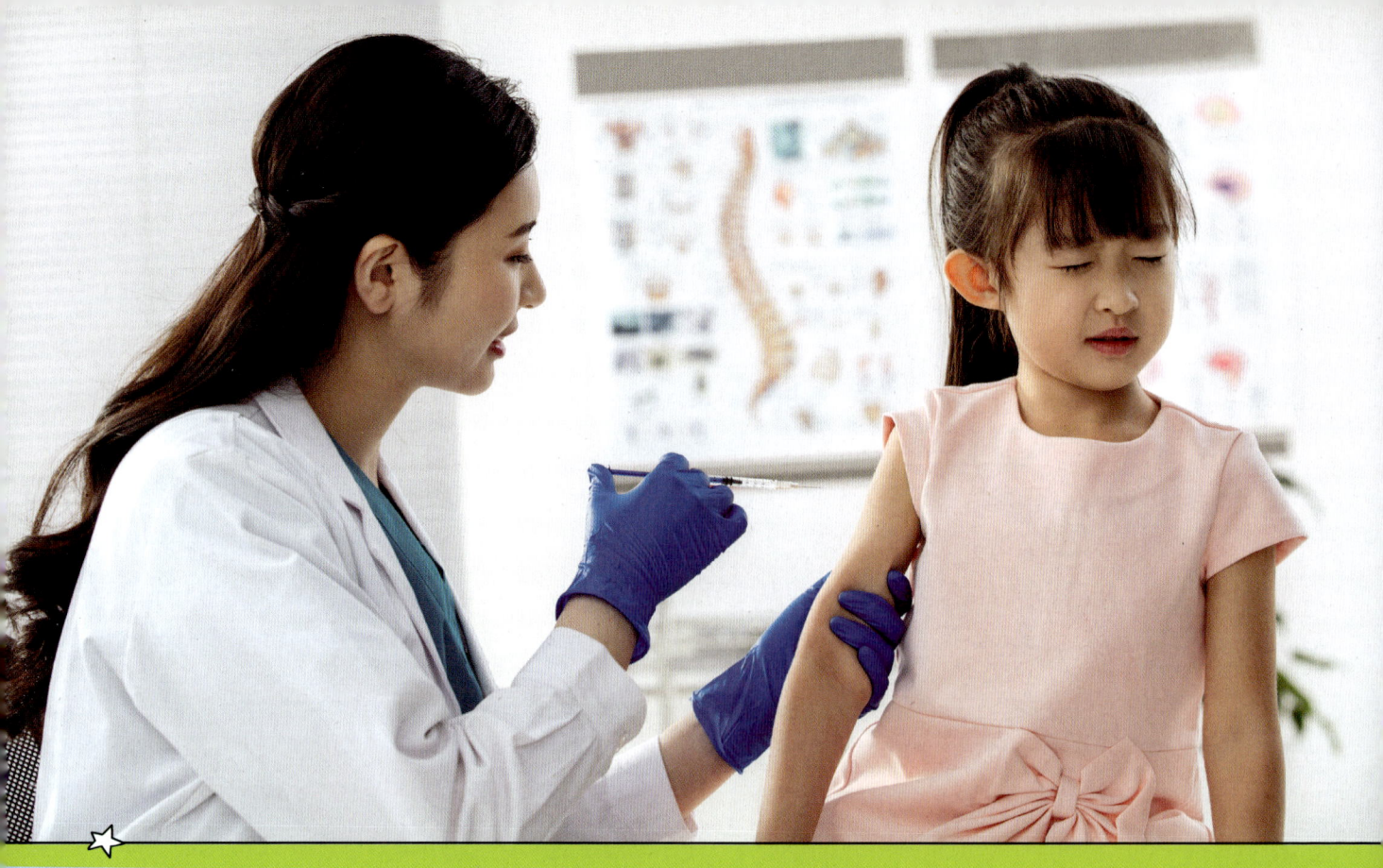

Some people do not like seeing the needle when they get an injection. You do not have to watch. You can look away. You can close your eyes. You never see the needle at all!

Being surprised by an injection is not pleasant either. Don't be afraid to speak up. Tell the nurse if you want to know exactly when it's going to happen.

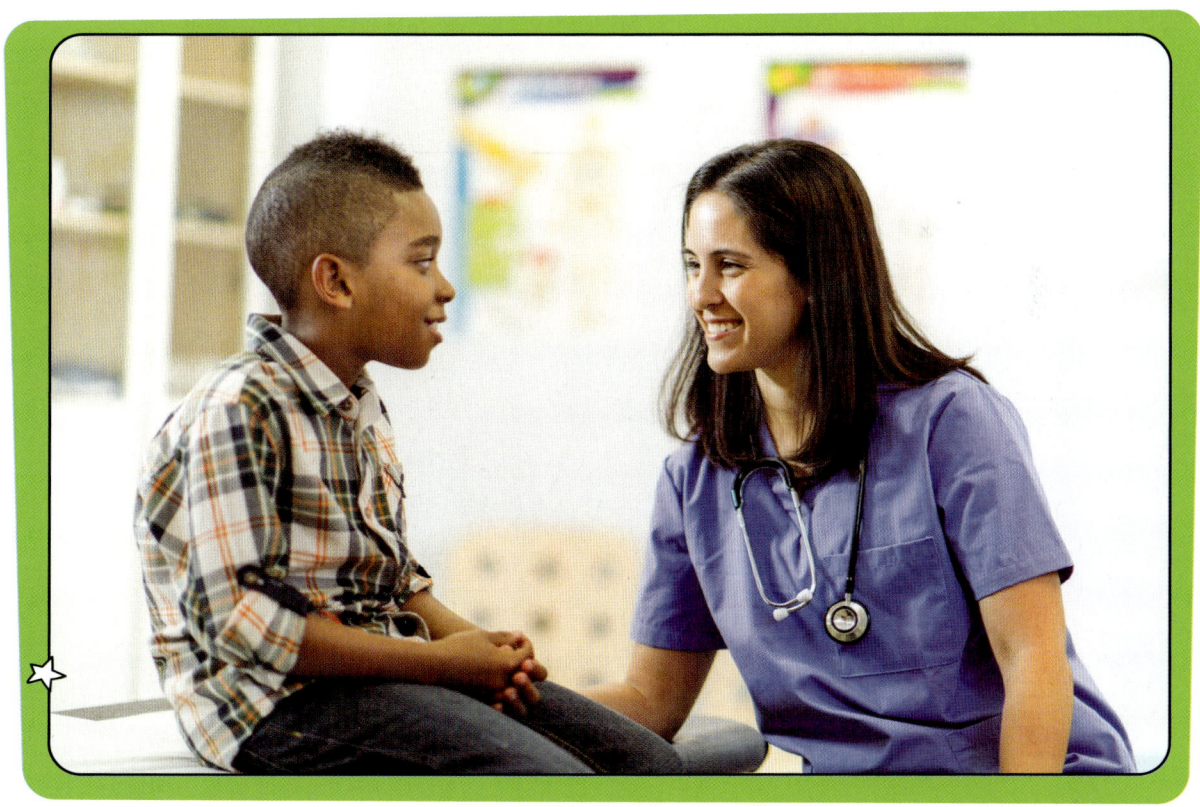

AFTER A VACCINATION

After a vaccination, your arm might feel **sore**. You might have **side effects**, such as a high temperature. This does not mean that you have an illness. You will feel better soon.

Tell an adult if you don't feel well. Rest and medicine can help.

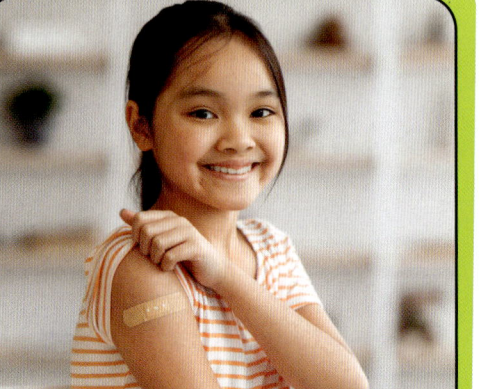

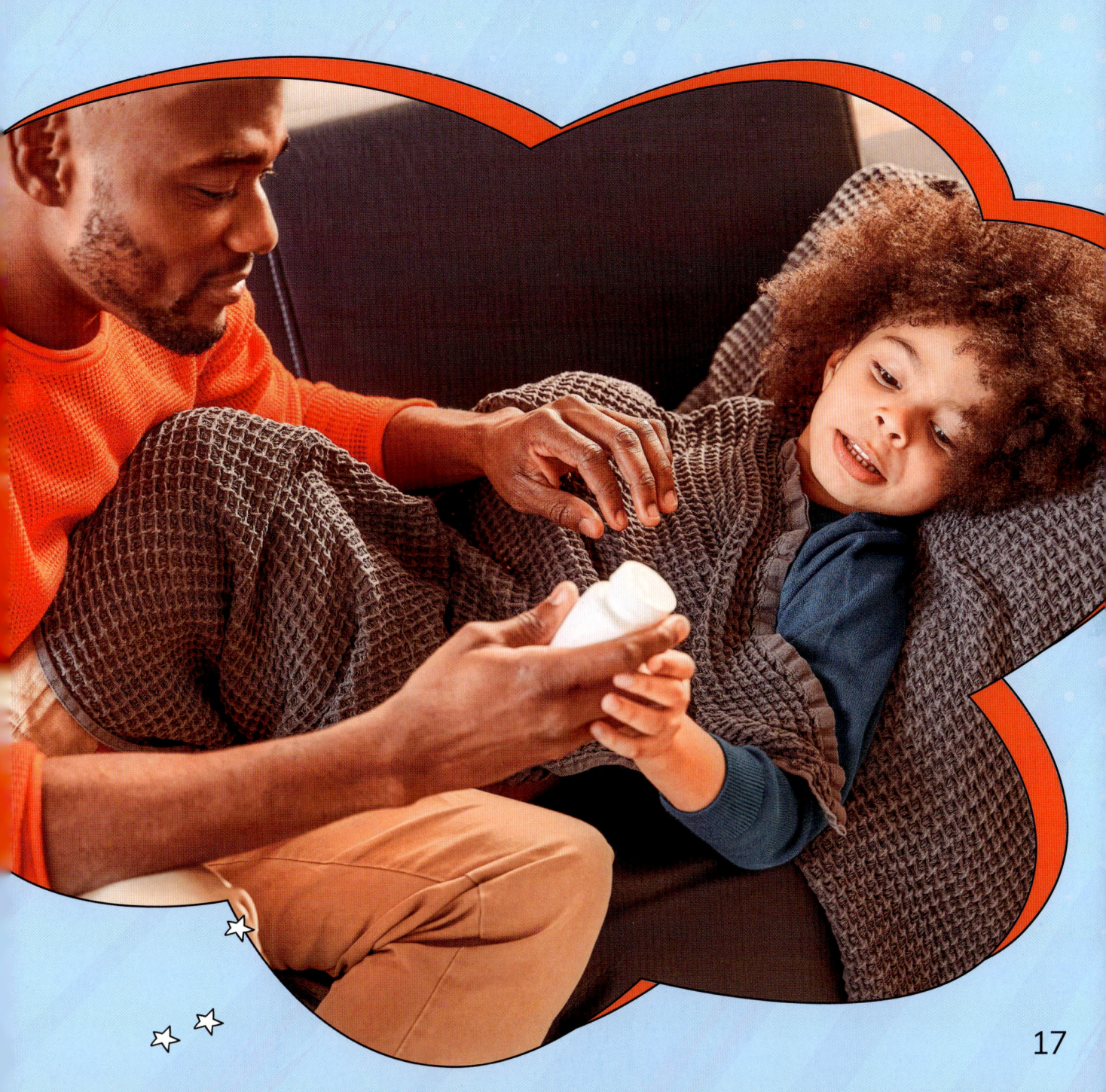

Getting a vaccination is not much fun. You probably won't ever learn to like it. But you can relax and get through it. Remind yourself that the injection is over in a flash.

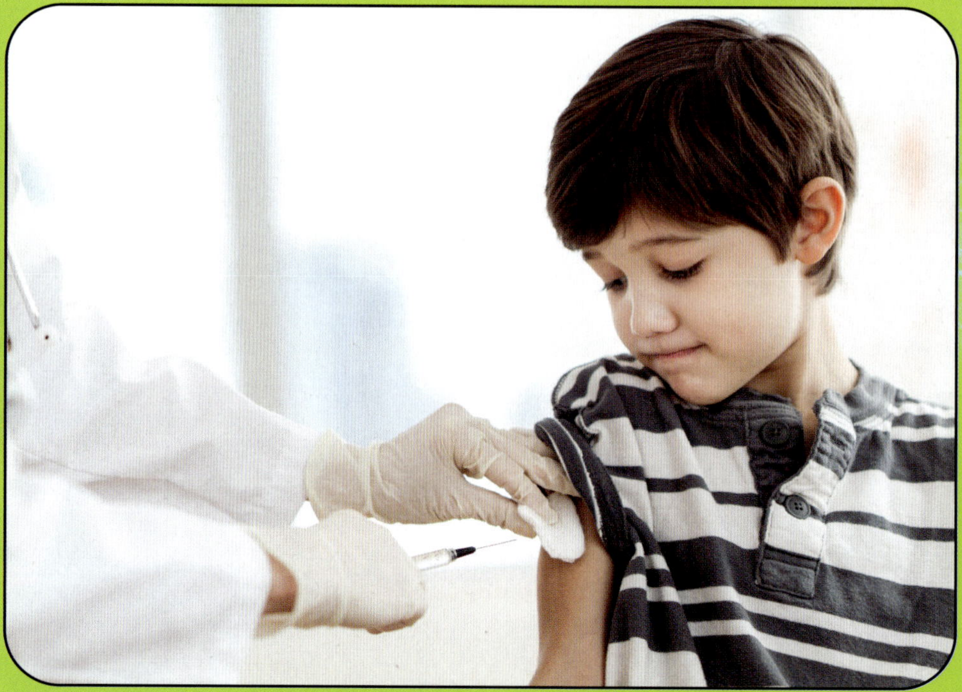

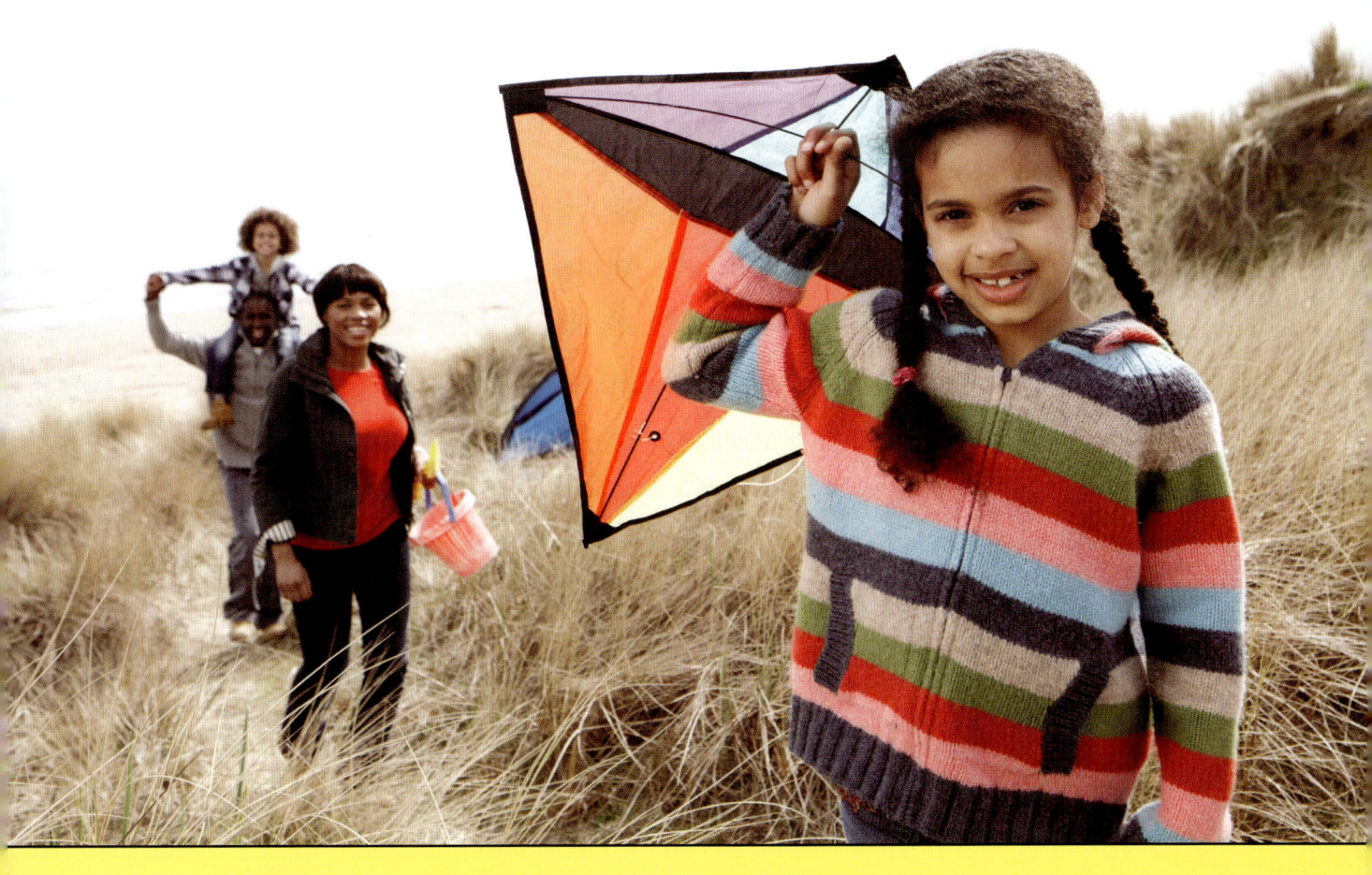

Remember how helpful vaccinations can be. They protect you and others around you from illness. That way, you can stay well and have some real fun!

HELP A FUZZY FRIEND

Pretend you are taking a toy animal to the doctor for a vaccination. Your fuzzy friend is scared. How can you help them to feel better?

What you need

- paper
- pencil
- toy animal

What to do

1. Think of one idea to relax before a vaccination.

2. Think of one idea to stay calm during a vaccination.

3. Think of one idea to feel better after a vaccination.

4. Write down all of your ideas.

5. Practise these ideas with your toy animal.

6. Then put your list of ideas in a safe place. Look at it the next time you need a vaccination!

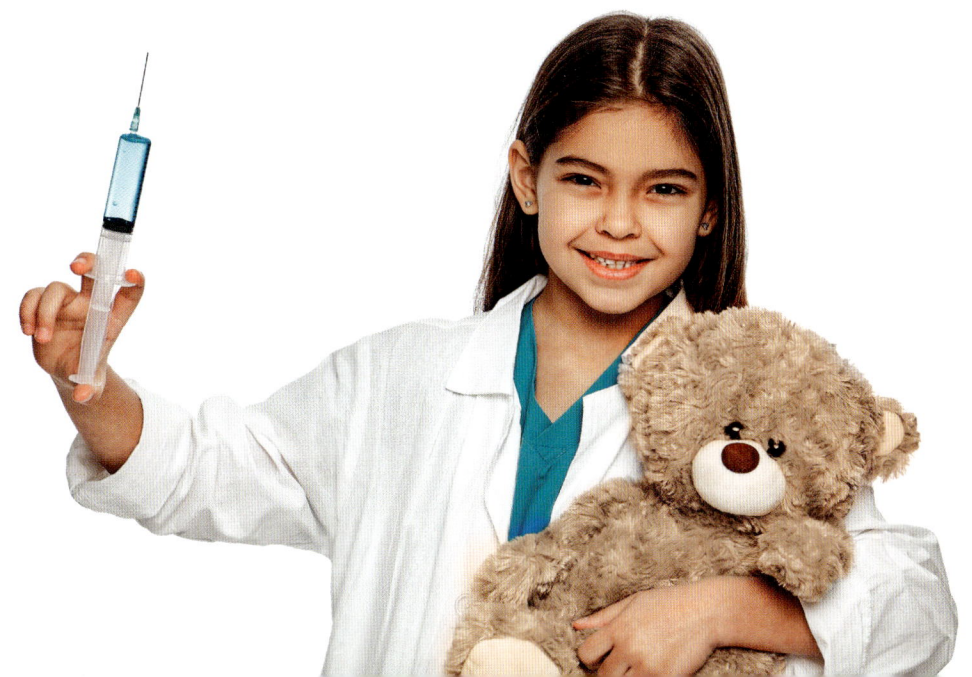

GLOSSARY

distract draw attention away from something

illness condition of being unhealthy in your body or mind

immune system system that protects your body from illness, infections and disease

side effect unwanted effect of a drug or chemical that occurs along with a desired effect

sore painful

vaccine substance that is usually injected into a person to protect against a particular disease

virus germ that infects living things and causes diseases. Viruses cause illnesses such as colds and flu.

FIND OUT MORE

BOOKS

All About Worries and Fears, Felicity Brooks (Usborne, 2022)

Human Body (DKfindout!), Bipasha Choudhury (DK Children, 2017)

My Mixed Emotions: Learn to love your feelings, Elinor Greenwood (DK Children, 2018)

WEBSITES

www.bbc.co.uk/newsround/51312915
Learn more about how vaccines work.

www.bbc.co.uk/bitesize/topics/zqbxqfr/articles/zqhbr82
Find out more about the parts of the human body.

INDEX

doctors 4

illness 6, 8, 16, 19

medicine 16

needles 10, 14

nurses 13, 15

pain 16

relaxing 12, 18

staying calm 4, 10

vaccines 8

ABOUT THE AUTHOR

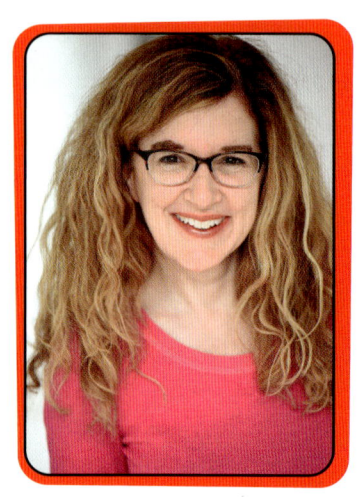

photo by Dan Doyle

Heather E. Schwartz has written hundreds of children's books. She lives in New York, USA, with her husband, two kids and two cats called Stampy and Squid. She often laughs when she feels scared, which helps her to calm down.